Being Female

Helen Farrer SRN, SCM

Richard J Doran MD
P Andrea Lum-Doran MD

Pitman Health Information Series

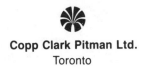

Copp Clark Pitman Ltd.
Toronto

First published in Australia
1980 by Pitman Publishing Pty Ltd
(second edition 1982)

ISBN 0-7730-4056-0

Design/Pauline McClenahan
Illustrations/Nan McNab
Typesetting/Q Composition Inc.
Printing and Binding/The Bryant Press Limited

Copp Clark Pitman Ltd.
495 Wellington Street West
Toronto, Ontario   M5V 1E9

Printed and bound in Canada

Contents

1
Being female

Being female has many delights, but all too often it has problems as well. This small book is written in the hope that the specifically female — gynecological — aspects of a woman's life might be better understood. It cannot delve very deeply into really rare conditions, but it does describe most of the common disorders, the ways of coping with them, and it tells when medical help should be sought.

What is normal?

Reproduction

Reproduction is what the whole system is designed to achieve. *Ovaries* produce ova (eggs), which, if fertilized, eventually grow into babies. The ovaries also produce chemical messengers — *hormones* — which travel through the bloodstream and prepare the *uterus* (womb) to receive these babies and also prepare the breasts to feed them. The uterus protects and provides for the *fetus* (unborn baby) and, at the end of pregnancy, it contracts to push it out into the world. The *vagina* provides a passage for sperm (from the male) to be deposited during

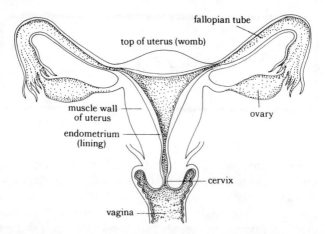

Figure 1.1 The internal reproductive organs (cross-section, viewed from behind)

intercourse, and a pathway through which the fetus is born. It also produces an acid moisture that prevents infection from gaining a hold in the vagina. Figures 1.1, 1.2, and 1.3 illustrate the female reproductive system.

Childhood

During childhood, the reproductive system is not actively functioning, and, apart from rare developmental disorders and infection (usually caused by self-exploration or very poor hygiene), there are no gynecological problems.

Puberty

At puberty the system awakens gradually, as the ovaries respond to hormonal messages from the pituitary gland.

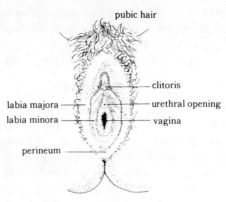

Figure 1.2 The vulva (external organs)

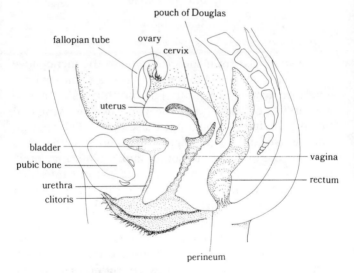

Figure 1.3 The pelvis, side view
(Source: M.M. Garrey et al, Obstetrics Illustrated, 2nd ed., Churchill Livingstone, Edinburgh, 1974, p 50)

The ovaries produce two hormones, *estrogen* and *progesterone*, which build up the lining of the uterus, make the vaginal moisture acid, cause the breasts to develop, and influence other feminine characteristics to appear.

Menarche

Menarche is the name given to the first menstrual period. The average age at which this happens is between twelve and thirteen years, but it can occur as early as ten years or as late as seventeen years and still be normal. If a girl reaches her eighteenth birthday without having started her periods, her doctor will order a full range of tests to find out the cause.

The reproductive years

These years last from the menarche to the menopause – from the first period to the last. (The age span is from about thirteen to about fifty.) If everything is normal, a woman will be fertile, that is capable of conceiving and having children, throughout these years. If she is sexually active, and having regular intercourse with a man without using some method of family planning, pregnancy will occur. The only times of natural infertility (apart from the infertile days in each cycle, which a woman can learn to recognize) are when a woman is already pregnant and after the menopause. A woman who is breast-feeding is only relatively infertile until the resumption of ovulatory menstruation occurs; therefore, some form of contraception excepting oral contraceptives is usually recommended during this period.

Ovulation

Once the reproductive system has organized itself (usually within the year following the first period) ovulation occurs regularly, approximately every four weeks (28 days). Ovulation is the release of an ovum by the ovary, from which it is quickly gathered up by the fallopian tubes and gently pushed towards the uterus. If the ovum encounters a sperm within twenty-four hours it will be fertilized, and a pregnancy will start. The fertilized ovum takes another seven or eight days to travel to the uterus, and, once there, it embeds and produces its own hormone, human chorionic gonadotropin (HCG), which prevents the lining of the uterus from breaking down.

Menstruation

If no pregnancy occurs, the prepared lining of the uterus disintegrates and comes away fourteen days after ovulation. Even in very irregular cycles, this figure (fourteen days) is usually constant. The average cycle, counted from the first day of bleeding to the first day of bleeding of the next period, is twenty-eight days. But anything from twenty-one days to thirty-five days can be regarded as normal, as long as the cycles are regularly short or long.

BLOOD LOSS

Blood loss is usually between 35 mL to 60 mL on the average with a maximum value of 100 mL, over about five days. It is usually moderate on the first day, heavier on the second day, and then it tapers off. Ten to fifteen pads or tampons should be adequate for any one period.

A normal flow should not soak through a securely fixed pad.

PERIOD PAIN

Some degree of pain and discomfort is usual during a period, especially on the first day or two. The uterus has to contract, its *cervix* (neck) has to open slightly and the small uterine blood vessels are in spasm. Really incapacitating pain is not normal and its cause should be discovered and treated (see dysmenorrhea, pages 17–18).

COPING WITH PERIODS

Mild to moderate discomfort can be helped by taking simple analgesics, e.g., A.S.A. – acetylsalicylic acid (Aspirin) or acetominophen (Tylenol), or by some of the tablets designed especially for the problem such as Midol. Heat applied to the abdomen often helps. For some women, it is worth lying down for an hour or so, when the discomfort is at its worst. Others find it better to keep moving; exercise, especially walking, improves the circulation and this may help to ease pelvic congestion. It is important to keep blood sugar levels high enough to cope during menstruation (especially on the first day of bleeding) by eating regular meals.

Normal vaginal discharge

Vaginal secretions are normally present and are increased at certain times during the menstrual cycle. The most important secretion occurs during the three or four days leading up to ovulation. This "ovulation" mucus is a clear, slippery, stretchy mucus that looks like raw egg-white, and it can be seen on the underwear or toilet paper. It comes from the glands in the cervix and is an important indicator of fertility. When ovulation occurs the mucus changes and becomes thick, and is not usually seen because it stays in the cervix and forms a protective plug.

Again, just before a period is due, it is normal to have a slight, cloudy discharge – this is the mucus secreted by glands in the lining of the uterus as it prepares to nourish a fertilized ovum.

Seminal fluid will also appear as a vaginal discharge for twelve to twenty-four hours following intercourse. It can resemble cervical (ovulation) mucus, but *abnormal* and infective discharges do not. Normal vaginal discharges are not profuse and do not have an unpleasant odour (see pages 9–10).

Pregnancy

Pregnancy is a normal happening in the female. It usually follows if intercourse occurs at, or close to, the time of ovulation. Sperm cells survive in the female for about three days, perhaps even longer in the presence of fertile mucus from the cervix. When conception occurs, usually in one of the fallopian tubes, the fertilized ovum is carried to the uterus where it implants. As mentioned earlier, it produces human chorionic gonadotropin (HCG), which is released into the mother's bloodstream. HCG keeps the ovary producing estrogen and progesterone, in enormous quantities. These hormones:

- Prevent the lining of the uterus from breaking down (so no period starts).
- Act on the breast (tingling and discomfort occur).
- Cause nausea and vomiting in some women.

Pregnancy tests, to examine the urine for the presence

of HCG, are carried out fourteen days after a period has been missed.

Menopause

The last menstrual period (*menopause*) occurs between the ages of forty-five and fifty-five years. It occurs because the ovaries simply age, and although they still contain egg cells (*ova*) they no longer respond to the hormonal messages from the pituitary gland. The production of estrogen and progesterone from the ovaries winds down and many of the changes that happened at puberty are now reversed. This process is called the *climacteric*, and it can cause many women to suffer unpleasant symptoms (see page 47).

2
Good gynecological health

Good gynecological health, like good dental health, requires a combination of good hygiene, prompt attention to symptoms, and regular checkups. As with the dentist, a lot of people are scared, embarrassed, or tolerate anything less than very severe symptoms and put off having regular checkups.

Hygiene

Good hygiene is a good preventive medicine. All it involves is regular (daily) washing of the body, including the vulva, changing the underwear every day, and laundering such things as towels and bed linen properly. It does not involve douching the vagina (except in very special circumstances) or spraying "feminine" deodorants on the vulva. Douches can upset the natural defences of the vagina and so make the woman susceptible to vaginal infections. Feminine sprays, despite their glossy advertisements and high prices, are unnecessary; in fact, they are a common cause of vulval and vaginal irritation, itching, and painful intercourse. The normal odour of the vaginal secretions is not offensive; on the contrary, it is one of the natural sexual stimulants in women. If the odour is bad, it is due either to poor hygiene, which can be corrected, or to a disorder, which should be investigated.

One aspect of hygiene that may not be known, yet is of great importance, concerns the direction of wiping the vulva after using the toilet, particularly after opening the bowels. If it is wiped from the back to the front (the easier arm action), the paper will carry bowel organisms forward along the vulva, from which they can enter the vagina. Many women have to learn and remember to deliberately wipe in the other direction, i.e., from front to back.

Symptoms that need urgent attention

Any of the following symptoms need urgent attention:
- Abnormal discharges or odours from the vagina.
- Abnormal or irregular bleeding.
- Bleeding following intercourse.
- Bleeding after the menopause.
- Persistent vulval itching.
- A lump on the vulva.
- A lump in the breast.

These are all discussed in more detail further on.

Gynecological checkups

No woman over the age of eighteen years (earlier if she is sexually active) can justify doing without regular gynecological examinations. They should be performed at least every two years during the reproductive years, and more often if there is a family history of gynecological cancer.

There are many "reasons" for putting off these check-ups — being too busy, not having any babysitters, not being able to get away from work, not being able to afford it, and there not being any symptoms. But the most common excuse is simply "hating going". Women hate going because they are shy, or embarrassed, or afraid to tell their symptoms to the doctor. Or they may fear that the examination will hurt or that something serious *will* be discovered.

An understanding doctor will help to overcome these fears, because he or she will know that they exist in so many people. If the doctor doesn't seem to understand or if he or she won't listen, then the woman should ask her friends to whom they go, or search until she can find a doctor with whom she can be confident and relaxed. It is so sad and foolish to neglect one's health, comfort, and happiness just because one doctor was abrupt, unsympathetic, disapproving, or not very gentle.

Most family doctors are experienced in routine gyne-cology, and most of them also understand when a woman asks to be referred to someone else, or to a gynecologist, for this aspect of her medical care. Most doctors appre-ciate the right of any patient to a second opinion.

Gynecological history

The first part of the checkup involves answering ques-tions, to give the doctor an outline of the woman's state of health and to discuss any symptoms that have arisen. On a first visit she will be asked:

- Her age, occupation, and marital status.
- Whether she has regular sexual activity and whether there are any problems with this.
- Her obstetric history – her pregnancies, babies born, and whether there were difficulties or complications.
- Her general health, medical history, and important family medical history.
- Whether she has ever had a blood transfusion.
- Whether she is taking any tablets (prescribed or otherwise) and whether she is having any other form of treatment currently.
- Whether she sleeps well.
- Whether there have been any significant recent personal events the doctor should know about.
- Whether she has any gynecological symptoms.

The questioning time is important both to the woman and to the doctor. On subsequent visits, the questions are usually confined to current symptoms and to any other matters that are bothering either of them.

The physical examination

Midway between periods is the best time for the examination. For the woman, it is less embarrassing and more comfortable than during menstruation or the days preceding it. For the doctor, it is easier to perform, allows a better assessment of the vagina and cervix, and enables him or her to check for the presence of ovulation mucus.

Before the examination, the woman is asked to remove

her panties and stockings, and to undo her bra. Any tight clothing which might get in the way is best taken off as well. The woman is usually given the opportunity to empty her bladder; the examination should not be painful, but it may be uncomfortable and isn't helped by a full bladder. The doctor or nurse will help the woman up on to an examination couch, will explain which way to lie, and will make sure that she is comfortable.

The first part of the examination is usually done with the woman in a relaxed sitting position commencing with an examination of her breasts. She will then be placed in a supine position (lying on her back). The

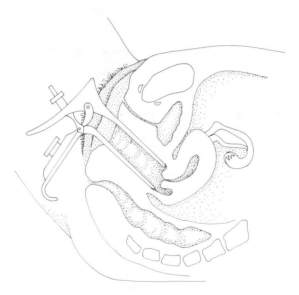

Figure 2.1 The speculum in position

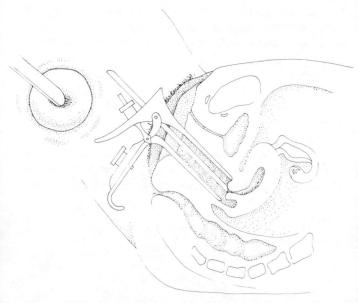

Figure 2.2 Obtaining a cervical smear

doctor will continue to examine her breasts and then the abdomen, looking and feeling for any abnormalities. The doctor may then instruct her to relax and place her in the lithotomy position (legs up in stirrups) or ask her to bring her knees up, heels together and to let her knees relax and flop sideways. After this the doctor will insert a lubricated instrument (a *speculum*) which helps to open out the vaginal walls and thus allows him or her to see the cervix (Figure 2.1). At this stage the doctor will take a "scraping" of cells from the cervix (the Papanicolaou smear test) to send away for testing for cervical cancer (Figure 2.2). If there is any unusual discharge from the cervix or the vagina the doctor will col-

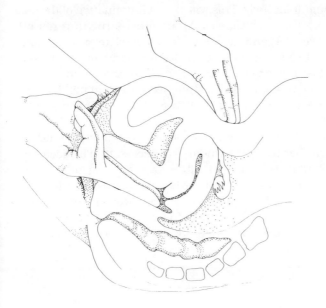

Figure 2.3 Bi-manual pelvic examination

lect some on a swab, to be tested for the presence of infection. Then the doctor will remove the speculum slowly, while noting the muscle tone of the vaginal walls.

The doctor then performs a bi-manual (two-handed) examination (see Figure 2.3), which allows him or her to feel the size and shape of the uterus and to note whether the ovaries feel normal. It is, however, the most uncomfortable part of the examination, because the ovaries are sensitive to pressure. Slow deep breathing, in and out, is a big help in keeping relaxed at this time. A rectovaginal examination is the insertion of a lubricated finger into the rectum and another into the vagina simultaneously. This will permit examination of the anal, rectovaginal wall, sacral, and other structures not otherwise felt and necessary for a complete examination.

After the examination, the woman can get dressed. Most doctors tell her not to hurry too much, because there is often a queer stretched sensation inside, and it may take a minute or two to go away. When she has dressed and tidied up, the woman will sit down with the doctor while he or she explains his or her findings and tells her if any treatments are necessary. The doctor will then advise her when she should come again.

The examination itself is usually over in a few minutes, and, having got it over, most women are really glad that they made the effort to go. And they are less reluctant to go again, when the next checkup is due.

3
Problems and symptoms

Painful periods – dysmenorrhoea

When the pain of a menstrual period is bad enough to interfere with daily life and it cannot be managed by using the simple measures suggested on page 6, a doctor's help should be sought. There are two, quite separate, types of dysmenorrhea – primary and secondary.

Primary dysmenorrhea

Dysmenorrhea is primary when there is no organic pathology (disease). It most often affects younger women and usually begins one or more years after menarche (onset of menstruation), and may be relieved by vaginal delivery of an infant or continue throughout the reproductive years gradually decreasing during the forties. The pain is sharp and cramping and is felt in the lower abdomen and back. It is worst during the first twelve hours after the period starts and may last for one to two days. It can be severe enough to cause fainting or vomitting.

It only occurs during ovulatory cycles and so one method of treatment is to suppress ovulation using the contraceptive "pill." Non-habit-forming pain-relieving drugs may be prescribed instead such as full doses of aspirin or acetominophen. The most effective treatment is the usage of anti-prostaglandin synthesis drugs. Prostaglandins are synthesized by the uterus and cause the main symptoms of dysmenorrhea. Drugs such as ibuprofen (Motin), mefenamic acid (Ponstel), and naproxen (Naprosyn, Anaprox) can alleviate the symptoms rapidly. In 15 per cent of the cases prostaglandin inhibitors do not succeed and temporary ovulation suppression may be tried with medical supervision. If all fails, *diagnostic laparoscopy* (visualization of internal organs with a scope) may be needed to establish unsuspected organic disease.

Secondary dysmenorrhea

Dysmenorrhea is termed secondary when the cause is attributed to a disease. Some diseases include endometriosis, pelvic inflammatory disease, uterine leiomyomas (fibroids), or adenomyosis.

It usually begins later than primary dysmenorrhea and sometimes even arises in the third and fourth decade. The pain can be premenstrual and comenstrual depending on the disease process.

Treatment is aimed at the cause, although symptomatic relief temporarily with analgesics or ovulation suppressors – "the pill" – may be given.

Pelvic Congestion

This is a different type of pain, rarely occurring before the mid-twenties. It is a "dragging," aching pain in the lower abdomen and upper thighs. It often comes on some days before the period starts, and may continue throughout the period, but usually begins to ease after the flow starts.

It is caused by congestion of the blood supply to the area, because of the increased amount supplying the uterus at this time, but there is usually some underlying disease or disorder as well. It can indicate chronic pelvic infection, endometriosis, or displacement of the uterus and so it should be investigated. Once the cause has been discovered it can usually be treated; the relief will be worth it. (Although some physicians still consider pelvic congestion to be a separate condition, others include this as secondary dysmenorrhea.)

Heavy periods – menorrhagia

The amount of blood lost during periods differs from woman to woman, but is usually not more than about 100 mL at the most. The body quickly replaces this small loss, well before the next period starts. Really heavy bleeding, however, may not be replaced quickly enough, and can leave the woman anemic, very tired, and susceptible to further ills.

If her periods are heavy, requiring more pads or tampons than they used to, last longer than they used to, or if they contain clots, the woman should seek medical help.

Menorrhagia is caused by infection of any of the internal pelvic organs (their blood supply increases to try to combat the infection), by fibroids, hormone imbalance, uterine cancer, endometriosis, intrauterine devices (IUDs), after several pregnancies, acute illnesses, anemia, and poor general health.

When the doctor is consulted about heavy periods he or she will do a full pelvic examination and will order a blood test to check the *hemoglobin* (iron) level. After that the doctor may decide to *curette* (scrape out) the lining of the uterus to examine the endometrium.

The treatment of heavy periods involves finding the cause and correcting it. Anemia is treated with courses of iron, sometimes by injection. Diet and lifestyle is looked at and may need to be adjusted to bring about the return of good health. If constipation is a problem, ways of correcting it will be worked out. Hormone imbalance may be treated by a carefully tailored prescription of estrogen and progestogen. Hysterectomy is performed in those cases where hormone therapy is unsuitable or where cancer, large fibroids, or endometriosis is present. Myomectomy removes large fibroids, while leaving the uterus intact for further pregnancies.

Missed periods – amenorrhea

There are many causes of missed periods, the commonest and most obvious being pregnancy. Amenorrhea also occurs naturally when a woman is fully breast-feeding and, of course, after the menopause.

Primary amenorrhea

In primary amenorrhea menstruation has never occurred. If a girl has not menstruated by the time of her eighteenth birthday, she should seek medical help. If she shows the other signs of puberty (breast development, pubic hair, etc.) it may be a relatively simple matter – that the hymen is imperforate. The *hymen* is a thin membrane which guards the entrance to the vagina and is the sign of physical virginity (it is broken with the first intercourse and almost completely disappears after childbirth). It does not completely close off the vagina; only rarely does it stretch right across and cut off the outlet, causing a build-up of old menstrual blood. Imperforate hymen is treated by simple incision, but it must be done in hospital with full antiseptic precautions.

Other causes of primary amenorrhea are the absence of the vagina, uterus, or ovaries, and pituitary or other glands and disorders.

Secondary amenorrhea

Secondary amenorrhea means that periods have occurred, but have stopped. The list of causes of unnatural amenorrhea is huge, and ranges from emotional upsets to brain tumours. It cannot be dealt with here, but amenorrhea is a symptom which should never be ignored. It should always be investigated, as it could be a sign of some disorder completely unconnected with the reproductive system.

Post-pill amenorrhea is becoming more common; it is caused by the continued suppression of the hormones that stimulate the ovaries. In some cases it is difficult to treat.

Premenstrual tension

This is a condition that can occur at any time during the latter half of the menstrual cycle (7 to 14 days before next menses). It is estimated to affect at least half of all women of child-bearing age. It also indirectly affects their husbands, children, and in fact, all their day-to-day relationships.

Premenstrual tension is believed to be the result of disturbed physiology. An increase in *aldosterone* (hormone for salt and water regulation) secretion by the adrenal gland has been implicated as the cause of water retention or *edema*. Imbalances between estrogen and progesterone have also been suggested as contributing factors, as well as psychologic factors. Some common symptoms are:

- Emotional instability, depression, headaches.
- Constipation, diarrhea.
- Abdominal swelling and discomfort, nausea, and vomiting.
- Swelling of the hands and feet.
- Breast enlargement and soreness.
- Poor physical co-ordination and clumsiness.

Treatment

Many doctors believe it is worthwhile seeing the woman and her husband together so that the doctor can explain the management of premenstrual tension to them. If the condition and its causes are understood, the family may be able to modify its lifestyle and reduce its physical and social demands on the woman during those days. This, along with the woman limiting her fluid intake and avoiding extra salt, will make the condition more manageable. Further medical treatment is aimed either at correcting the hormonal imbalance or at reducing the water retention.

The "pill" may be prescribed or, instead, progestogen alone can be beneficial in some cases. *Diuretics*, drugs which remove water from the tissues and cause it to be passed with the urine, are often successful. They are best begun before the symptoms are expected to arise and continued throughout the period. There are many different diuretic agents available, and the usage of these pills should be under medical supervision.

Vaginal discharges

Abnormal discharges are usually due to an infection. They may come from the uterus, from the cervix, or, most commonly, from the vagina. Normally the vagina is resistant to infection because of the acidity of its secretions, and because it is inhabited by microscopic "friendly" organisms – *lactobacilli* – that attack most invading organisms and keep their numbers under control. Both vaginal acidity and lactobacilli are dependent on the presence of estrogen. Estrogen deficiency vaginitis causes a thin, grey-yellow, irritating discharge and is due to a variety of organisms multiplying in the absence of the natural defences. It is treated by estrogen tablets (in low doses) or by local application of estrogen creams. Acid vaginal jelly or yoghurt (applied each night into the vagina) may be used instead, when estrogen is not advised.

Monilia (thrush)

Monilia causes a thick white cheesy discharge, not profuse but very irritating. It is caused by a fungus, *Candida albicans*, which is often a normal inhabitant of the vagina but which is kept under control by the lactobacilli. However, the most intense symptom is *vulvar pruritus* (itch) followed by vaginal burning, *dyspareunia* (painful intercourse), and *dysuria* (painful urination). Thrush can be troublesome:

- During, and just after, menstruation (blood in the vagina affects the acidity levels).
- In pregnancy, when on the "pill," and in diabetics – all states in which increased sugar is present (on which the fungi thrive).
- When taking antibiotics which kill the lactobacilli.

It is made worse by tight synthetic underwear and poor hygiene, and therefore meticulous hygiene is a must as well as cotton underwear.

As infection can be sexually spread the sexual partner's history of pertinent symptoms must be sought. Treatment can be local or systemic and aimed at one or both partners. Some local antifungal agents are mycostatin (Nystatin), chlortrimazol (Canestan or Mycolog), and miconazde nitrate (Monistat). Oral mycostatin can be given in conjunction with local vaginal and/or penile treatment.

Trichomonas vaginalis

Trichomonal infection causes a profuse yellow frothy discharge that is foul-smelling and irritating. It is usually spread by sexual intercourse but not in every case – occasionally it may be spread by towels, water, or toilet seats.

Treatment is by taking metronidazole (Flagyl) by mouth. The husband (or sexual partner) should also be treated to prevent reinfection. Extra care with bathing and laundering is advised. Treatment may take up to six weeks to clear trichomonal infections and for that time sexual intercourse should be avoided.

Gonorrhea

Gonorrhea causes a yellow discharge, which may be profuse or mild. The other signs of gonorrhea are frequency and burning on passing urine, and vulval soreness. Gonorrhea is the most common infectious disease in Canada today.

Treatment is by large doses of penicillin by injection or other antibiotics such as Ampicillin with probenecid or tetracycline. Because antibiotics are so easy to obtain, self-treatment is sometimes practised. This may be sufficient to control the symptoms but not to kill all the infecting organisms, and sexual partners are often not treated. To be sure of overcoming the disease and avoiding complications, *medical* help from a doctor or clinic must be sought *immediately.*

If the symptoms are mild, or ignored, and gonorrhea is not treated properly, it can spread through the reproductive system and invade the fallopian tubes, causing inflammation, adhesions, and, ultimately, sterility.

Other causes of vaginal discharge are:

- Forgotten tampons.
- Irritating douches.
- Chronic infection of the cervix.
- Following certain operations on the vagina or cervix.
- Intrauterine devices (sometimes).
- *Herpes simplex* infection.
- Cancer of the cervix (often not until the growth is well advanced).

All abnormal discharges ought to be investigated so that their causes can be treated. Some are very unpleasant to live with and demand relief. Others, such as *Herpes simplex* and cancer of the cervix have mild symptoms, that seem to matter little, but they could be the first indication of very serious disease.

Itching and scratching

Pruritus (itching) of the vulva is a common and miserable symptom. If it is not cleared up it can become chronic and very difficult to treat. Itching leads to scratching, which causes skin damage, and the damaged skin is irritative and itchy – a vicious cycle. Chronic pruritus is sometimes a forerunner of vulval cancer – a condition requiring extensive surgery.

Causes

Causes of itching include:

- Irritation from vaginal discharges.
- Urine left on the skin.
- Allergies to chemicals in drugs, soaps, vaginal deodorants, and contraceptives.
- Tight or synthetic underclothing.
- General diseases, especially diabetes.
- Poor dietary or hygiene habits.
- Cancer of the vulva.
- Emotional factors.

Emotional factors can work by themselves – many people feel itchy when they see another person scratching. Even just talking or thinking about itchiness can set them off. But usually the emotional factors appear in combination with a physical cause, making that cause seem more obvious.

Things that make itching worse are warmth, anxiety, worry, and tiredness. So it is in bed, at night, that it is at its worst, and it is here that scratching often happens, perhaps even unconsciously.

Treatment

Local treatment is generally useless if the real cause is not treated. So all itching that does not respond to good and careful hygiene must be investigated by a doctor. The simpler causes are eliminated first and a general physical examination is made. After this, special tests for diabetes, blood disorders, and allergies may be ordered. Where cancer of the vulva is suspected (it is rare, but possible), a skin biopsy is carried out.

Once diagnosed, the cause is treated. But, for a full cure, the itching cycle must be stopped and the damaged skin must heal. So the things that can make the itching worse, that are in addition to the basic cause, are discussed. Electric blankets might be the problem. Cool baths are better than hot showers; they stimulate the skin less. Soap is best not used until the itch has gone, and then only very mild, non-perfumed soap. Vaginal deodorants, douches, chemical contraceptives, and laundry powders are discussed. The wearing of synthetic underwear and tight jeans is advised against, the best underwear being ones made from 100 per cent cotton. Planning the woman's day well, to avoid becoming overtired, and relaxing before going to bed to ensure a good night's sleep, will help. Cotton gloves worn in bed (and, of course, keeping the fingernails short) will lessen the risk of skin damage.

CONTROLLING THE URGE TO SCRATCH
Local applications of soothing powders such as zinc and starch powder dusted on lightly, or lotions such as cal-

amine, often help. Patent "cures" may make things worse, and are best avoided. Prescribed creams should be used regularly and kept close at hand, so that they can be applied as soon as itching occurs. Firm pressure over the itching area will often stop the itching.

OTHER MEASURES INCLUDE:

- A good diet for proper healing.
- Exposing the area to light and air (but not heat).
- Sometimes antibiotics, to prevent infection.

Pruritus which refuses to clear despite every effort to control it is known as *intractable pruritus.* In such a case the woman may have no relief from the itching until the skin of the area is removed by the operation of simple vulvectomy.

Urinary problems

Special problems arise in women because the urinary system is so closely related to the reproductive system. It is really important to have urinary problems diagnosed and treated because, if they become chronic, they could lead to serious kidney or other medical diseases.

Frequency

Normally the bladder sends signals to the brain only when it is becoming full, but, when it or the urethra is irritated, it signals earlier and more often. This is caused by:

- Pressure on the bladder – from a pregnancy, a pelvic tumour, or tight clothing.

- Infections of the vulva, vagina, urethra, or bladder.
- Too much urine, from too much fluid drunk, or as in some medical and renal conditions.
- The "psychogenic bladder" – nervousness and never being able to pass a toilet without "going."

Incontinence

STRESS INCONTINENCE

Stress incontinence is due to lax bladder supports, especially weakness of the bladder neck, which won't stay closed under any increased pressure. When the woman laughs or coughs or sneezes, urine runs away without warning. Stress incontinence is most common in women who have had children and who are at, or past, the menopause. It is worse if they are overweight or have a chronic cough (such as a chronic smoker's cough). It is treated by physiotherapy – exercises to tone up the pelvic floor – or, more commonly, helped by surgery – by vaginal repair or urethral suspension operation (see page 64).

URGENCY INCONTINENCE

Urgency incontinence is different. There is a warning, but the warning is almost immediately followed by strong bladder contractions that push the urine out. It is caused by bladder irritability and often responds well to anti-spasmodic drugs, which reduce the force of the bladder muscle contractions.

TRUE INCONTINENCE

True incontinence is a lot less common. Urine dribbles away continually because of a *fistula* (hole) between the bladder or urethra and the uterus or vagina. It used to happen after a long obstructed labour, but that is rare today. Nowadays its main causes are invasive cancer, radiation treatment, and damage during pelvic operations.

Continuous dribbling of urine causes discomfort and infection. True incontinence is treated by draining the bladder through a tube (*catheter*) until either natural healing has occurred or any infection has cleared enough to repair the fistula safely by operation.

"Honeymoon cystitis"

Also called the urethral syndrome, "honeymoon cystitis" is a chronic condition with very acute urinary symptoms of frequency, pain, and burning. The pain may be so bad that urinating is impossible except when in a warm bath. It affects only some women, and there is no way of knowing who will be susceptible. Once it starts it can take months or even years to clear up. It is caused by damage to the short sensitive urethra during intercourse. Also, bacteria may be pushed into the urethra during intercourse, and may establish chronic infection.

The symptoms usually do not appear until about thirty-six hours after intercourse, and so the connection may not be realized. But unless the condition is recognized and managed well, it can have serious effects. Intercourse will not be welcome when the symptoms are present because the area hurts so much, and it will not be welcome later if it is going to start the whole business off again.

The doctor will order an examination of a midstream specimen of urine to try to identify the infection and prescribe suitable antibiotics. Often, however, the test is negative or shows only a very mild infection, yet the symptoms are very severe. Even so, a lot of relief can be obtained by following the suggestions below:

- Double (for a while at least) the daily fluid intake. This will make the urine a lot weaker and less acidic.

- Empty the bladder immediately before and (especially) after intercourse, to flush out any organisms that might have been introduced before they gain a hold in the urethra.

- Drink two glasses of water immediately after inter-course.

4
Sexuality

With changing cultural attitudes, the former premarital counselling on sexuality, reproduction, and other gynecologic questions are now being posed by women of all ages including young girls. The latter two are discussed in other sections of this book leaving the enormous topic of sexuality to be dealt with here.

The normal female sexual response biologically is divided into four stages. *Stage I – Excitement* includes vaginal congestion, enlargement, and lubrication; increased heart rate, blood pressure, and respiratory rate; nipple erection and increase of breast volume. *Stage II – Plateau* consists of maximal vaginal swelling and coloration of labia minora (see Figure 1.2), uterine ascension and clitoris rotation and retraction. *Stage III – Orgasm* is the reflex rhythmic contractions of circumvaginal and pelvic floor muscles. Clitoral stimulation during foreplay is important for climax. *Stage IV – Resolution* is the resumption of the genitalia to non-aroused state.

Masturbation is considered to be a healthy and normal form of sexual activity. There are many other sexual techniques, including a vast number of coital positions, and further information can be obtained from the physician. The area of homosexuality also poses many questions outside the scope of this book.

Inhibited Sexual Desire

This is a clinical syndrome in which there is an absence or low desire for sexual activity with no arousal feelings even after stimulation although lubrication and climax may occur but with minimal pleasure. The most common cause is depression often accompanied by sleep and eating disturbances. Stress, drugs, hormones, and psychological factors can also result in decreased sexual desire.

Pain with intercourse – dyspareunia

This is a distressing symptom and one which many people find difficult to discuss. Pain may be superficial or deep. Superficial dyspareunia is felt at the entrance to the vagina, whereas deep dyspareunia is felt inside the pelvis and may last for some hours after intercourse.

Superficial dyspareunia

Superficial pain may be caused by:

- Tenderness of the vulva, urethra, or vagina due to infection or allergic reactions.
- Hemorrhoids.
- Dryness, caused by douching or the absence of estrogen (after the menopause).
- Tightness of the vaginal opening, due to a thick hy-

men or following scarring after childbirth or operations.

Deep dyspareunia

Deep pain may be caused by:

- Tenderness in the pelvis due to endometriosis, pelvic infection, or tumours.
- Displacements of the uterus, retroversion, or prolapse.
- Scar tissue in the upper vagina following operation or radiation.
- Psychological factors.

PSYCHOLOGICAL FACTORS

Psychological factors include: mental attitude to sex, previous bad experiences, lack of privacy, worries, tiredness, fear of pregnancy and labour, and lack of education or explanation following gynecological operations or childbirth.

Vaginismus

Vaginismus is muscle spasm of the pelvic floor, causing the vagina to close tightly, making intercourse impossible. Sometimes the muscles of the thigh also go into spasm and it is impossible for the woman even to open her legs. The spasms cause sharp shooting pains that are very distressing. Vaginismus is due to the pain or the fear of pain with intercourse.

Treatment of dyspareunia

Unless the cause is simple and obvious, the woman should seek the advice of a doctor with whom she can discuss the problem. She will need a gently-performed pelvic examination, perhaps under a general anesthetic if it is too painful.

Lubricants may be advised for simple dryness, estrogen by mouth or as a cream for post-menopausal dryness, or an acid lubricating jelly if estrogen is not suitable. Tightness may be relieved by gentle stretching, or by vaginal dilators, or by simple surgery.

Psychological causes and vaginismus are more difficult for a general practitioner or general gynecologist to treat. They will, however, refer the couple to a specialist in sexual medicine if matters don't improve after a short time. The treatment and counselling given by such specialists is usually very effective in resolving the condition.

Abstinence from intercourse is often recommended during the period of investigation and treatment. If intercourse is attempted before the problems have been solved, dyspareunia will probably return and may even be worse than before.

5
Gynecological disorders

Endometriosis

Endometriosis is a condition in which deposits of *en-dometrium* (the lining of the uterus) are growing in the wrong places. They may grow on the ovaries, throughout the pelvic cavity, in the pouch of Douglas (see Figure 1.2 page 3), on the bladder, and on the bowel. Occasionally they are seen in the navel and in operation scars.

Its precise cause is not known, but it may be due to *retrograde menstruation* – the uterine contractions forcing particles of endometrium out through the tubes so that they drop into the pelvic cavity. Endometriosis can also be spread during operations on the uterus or other pelvic surgery, and via the bloodstream.

The deposits undergo the same building-up and breaking-down process as does the uterine lining during the menstrual cycle, but there is no escape route for the bleeding, and so it gathers and forms cysts. These cysts, because of their content – dark, tarry, half-absorbed old blood – are called "chocolate cysts." They sometimes rupture and cause pelvic adhesions and *peritonitis* (inflammation).

Symptoms

Symptoms are dysmenorrhea, abnormal uterine bleed-ing, painful intercourse, infertility, and bowel and blad-

der problems, depending on where the deposits are. When
they are on the surface of the vagina or the skin (navel
or operation scars) they are extremely painful if touched.

Treatment

Diagnosis is made after pelvic examination and sometimes laparoscopy (see page 66). Treatment should be
based on the severity of the disease, age of patient, and
intention of childbearing. In general, mild cases can be
treated with exogenous hormones (Danazol, estrogen,
and progesterone) with surgery for moderate to severe
cases. If reproduction is still desired, conservative surgery alone or with a prior course of Danazol for 3–6
months is recommended. If the symptoms are really bad,
a *hysterectomy* (removal of the uterus) with removal of
the ovaries as well is performed.

Fibroids

Fibroids are non-malignant growths of fibrous and muscle tissue within the walls of the uterus. They are very
common, grow slowly, and vary in size from that of a
small seed to that of a large grapefruit. They depend on
estrogen for their growth and usually shrink after the
menopause.

Symptoms

Symptoms depend on the number and size of the fibroids. Large ones can cause very heavy periods (and
anemia), pressure on the bowel or bladder, backache,
and infertility. They can be a problem in pregnancy (if
the woman *becomes* pregnant) by causing miscarriage,
premature labour, or obstruction of the birth canal.

Treatment

Iron is given for anemia, so that the woman is well enough for surgery. *Myomectomy*, removal of the fibroids alone, is carried out if the uterus is to be saved for childbearing, otherwise the best treatment for fibroids causing severe symptoms is hysterectomy.

Ovarian cysts

These are growths arising in the ovary. They may be solid or filled with fluid, and either type may be benign or malignant. They can form at any age. There are literally dozens of types of ovarian cyst and so no attempt will be made to list them here. The important fact to note is that many of these growths are symptom-free for a long time. They may grow quite large, but, because the ovary is insensitive to stretch, pain is usually absent. Abdominal enlargement can be blamed on "middle-age spread" or to overeating.

Pain does occur at times, but this is usually associated with complications such as infection, adhesions, rupture, or twisting. Symptomless ovarian cysts are often discovered during a routine gynecological checkup. As several of the benign cysts can become malignant it is important that they be discovered and treated appropriately according to the type of cyst.

Malignant tumours

Malignant tumours can occur in the vulva, cervix, endometrium, and the ovaries, and, more rarely, in the vagina and fallopian tubes.

Vulval cancer

Vulval cancer may first be felt as a painless lump – perhaps only discovered during a routine gynecological examination – or it may arise after many years of vulval irritation (pruritus). It is treated by a radical vulvectomy operation, which removes the whole of the vulval skin and underlying fat, and the pelvic lymph glands.

Cervical cancer

Cervical cancer is the second most common cancer in women; breast cancer being more common. Those most at risk are women:

- Between ages of eighteen and thirty-five and have had sexual intercourse.
- Who have had early intercourse.
- Who have had multiple sexual partners.
- Who have had chronic cervical and vaginal infections.
- Who have poor personal hygiene.

SYMPTOMS

Symptoms appear late, unfortunately. In order to discover the disease before it becomes invasive, all women who are sexually active should have Papanicolaou smear tests annually. The classic signs not to be ignored, are abnormal or unusual bleeding, particularly following intercourse, and a watery brown discharge. Positive smears are always repeated, to check that there had been no errors in collection or handling. If suspicious cells are discovered on the repeat smear, a punch biopsy may be performed or a cone-shaped wedge of the cervix may be removed (a cone excision).

TREATMENT

Treatment of cervical cancer depends on the degree of spread. Surgical removal of all reproductive organs (cervix, uterus, ovaries, upper vagina) with or without concomittant removal of pelvic lymph glands may be necessary (Wertheim's hysterectomy). Radiation therapy can also be used alone or together with surgery depending on the stage. Although survival rates are improving, there are still many preventable fatal cases of cervical cancer.

Endometrial cancer

Cancer of the uterus is less common than cervical cancer, and is found in an older age group, usually between fifty-five and sixty-five years. It tends to be hereditary, and occurs more commonly in women who are significantly overweight or who have high blood pressure or diabetes.

The first sign is irregular or unusual bleeding, and any post-menopausal woman with that sign must seek help immediately. She will most likely need to have a curettage of the uterus to exclude cancer. The treatment for endometrial cancer is by hysterectomy (removal of uterus, ovaries, cervix, and pelvic lymphadenectomy), by irradiation, or by very high doses of progestogen, whichever is more suitable for the extent of the cancer.

Prolapses

Prolapse means "falling down" and in gynecology it refers to the uterus or the vaginal walls coming into the vagina, because their normal supports have weakened.

Prolapse is most common in women who have had children, and who have reached the menopause. Childbirth puts a great strain on the ligaments and pelvic floor, and estrogen withdrawal causes the pelvic tissues and vaginal walls to become devitalized.

When the supports fail, the uterus will descend, and it will drag with it the upper vaginal walls. This upsets the normal support of the bladder and the rectum. Prolapse of the bladder wall is called *cystocele*; prolapse of the rectal wall is called *rectocele*.

Symptoms

These may be:

- A dragging pain and backache, due to tension on the uterine ligaments, if the prolapse is mild. Where the uterus has completely prolapsed and lies outside the vulva, the ligaments have completely given up resistance, and so there is less tension.

- A feeling of something coming down, or a lump in the vagina.

- Urinary symptoms, especially frequency, stress incontinence, and inability to empty the bladder completely. With cystocele, some of the bladder lies below the level of the bladder neck. Unless it is lifted up via the vagina, the urine in that part of the bladder cannot be passed. Many women learn to do this instinctively, but are often too shy to mention it to a doctor.

- Bowel symptoms. With rectocele, there is often constipation and incomplete emptying of the rectum. As with cystocele, it may be necessary to support the prolapsed vaginal wall to empty the bowels properly.

Treatment

Prolapses are usually treated only if they are causing symptoms.

SUPPORTING PESSARIES

A vinyl ring is placed at the top of the vagina to hold out the walls and so prevent the uterus from falling down. It is used rarely today, and usually for women who are too old or sick to have surgery.

OPERATIONS

Vaginal repair operations, *colporrhaphy*, strengthen the vaginal walls. *Perineorrhaphy* repairs a lax perineum. *Manchester repair* includes removal of some of the cervix to lessen strain on the uterine ligaments. Sling operations such as the *Marshall-Marchetti procedure* are also often used.

Vaginal hysterectomy and repair – removal of the uterus via the vagina and repair of the vaginal walls – is done for a completely prolapsed uterus, or when there is a lesser prolapse but when there is some other reason to remove the uterus, for example, if the periods are very heavy.

Retroversion

Retroversion means that the uterus is tilted backwards. It can be due to lax ligaments in the months following childbirth or to some other pelvic condition. Growths such as fibroids and cysts may push the uterus backwards; adhesions or endometriosis may pull the uterus backwards.

Symptoms

Sometimes there are none, otherwise retroversion may cause:

- Backache.
- Painful periods.
- Painful intercourse.
- Infertility.

Treatment

Retroversion discovered incidentally (a routine examination) and which is causing no symptoms, is not treated and has no detrimental effects. However, the specific treatment must be directed at the cause – fibroids, cysts, adhesions, etc. If no organic cause is found with persistent symptoms, an operation to hold the uterus forward (*ventrosuspension*) may be advised.

Infertility

Infertility can be defined as the inability of a couple to conceive and continue the pregnancy with eventual delivery of a live birth. Infertility is not uncommon; it happens in about 10 per cent of marriages, and it can happen to people who have already had children.

Reasons for infertility

Unless the five factors necessary for conception (see Figure 5.1) are present, pregnancy will not occur.

MALE PROBLEMS

Male problems, relating to the number or quality of sperm. can be caused by hormone disorders, undescended tes-

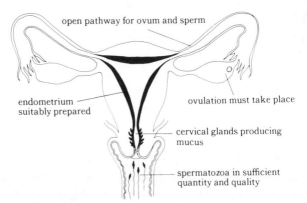

Figure 5.1 Factors necessary for conception

ticles, mumps after puberty, certain drugs, chronic infection, excessive warmth near the testes, overtiredness, and heavy drinking and smoking.

FEMALE PROBLEMS
Female problems include not ovulating (due to hormone imbalance, post-pill infertility, or certain drugs), and not having intercourse at the time of ovulation. Cervical mucus might be absent following treatment such as cauterization to the cervix. Obstruction of the fallopian tubes can occur following gonorrhea, tuberculosis, or other infections. Adhesions from operations, endometriosis, or infections can distort the tubes or cause their ends to close. The lining of the uterus can be affected by hormonal disorders, endometriosis, fibroids, foreign bodies (e.g., the IUD), and infection.

MALE AND FEMALE PROBLEMS
Problems in both can include: general ill health, anemia, overwork; psychological problems, even minor ones,

which can then be made worse by the infertility itself — "trying too hard," immunity to a particular man's sperm by a particular woman's body.

Investigations

The woman usually seeks help first and has a general physical and gynecological examination that confirms or rules out obvious causes. After this, the man is asked to provide a specimen of *semen* (the sperm-containing fluid ejaculated during intercourse) to be analysed. Alternatively, the woman undergoes examination as soon as possible after intercourse (*Huhner's test*) to see whether the sperm in and around the cervix are normal in quality and quantity.

If the sperm tests are satisfactory, the fallopian tubes are checked for blockages, either by X ray (*hysterosalpingogram*) or by air pressure (*Rubin's test*). If the tubes are normal the doctor may order a curette to examine the endometrium or a laparoscopy to examine the pelvis under direct vision. Curettage and laparoscopy both require admission to hospital for a day or two.

Psychological causes are harder to investigate. Sometimes they require the services of a specialist in psychosomatic gynecology or sexual medicine. Often, however, the simple fact that "something is being done at last" about the infertility has very positive effects.

New developments

New developments in infertility treatment have given hope to many childless couples. Microsurgery has enabled damaged fallopian tubes to be repaired. Artificial insemination techniques using sperm donated from husband or donor have been used with success. One technique for removing the ovum from the woman's body, fertilizing it outside, and then placing it in the woman's prepared uterus has been successful, and has produced the world's first "test-tube babies." Continuing research into natural family planning (the ovulation mucus method) is being documented by scientific evidence, and is contributing much to the study of fertility and infertility.

6
Menopausal problems

The *climacteric* or "change of life" is, although a normal process, in fact a state of hormonal deficiency. In some women it happens gradually, with slight symptoms, and can be coped with easily. In others it is abrupt, with severe symptoms, and it can cause much physical and emotional misery. The symptoms are due either to a lack of estrogen or to a rise in the pituitary hormones in response to low estrogen levels.

Symptoms

Symptoms may include any of the following:
- Menstruation stops, often after irregular, infrequent periods, sometimes light, sometimes heavy.
- The vulva and vagina lose tone, become dryer, and are less resistant to infection. Intercourse may become difficult and vaginal discharge and itching may arise.
- Pelvic supports lose tone, and prolapse and urinary problems can occur.
- Pituitary overactivity may cause changes in the blood vessels, resulting in hot flushes, palpitations, and headaches.

- Associated problems of anxiety, depression, fatigue, and loss of sleep.

Management

As the climacteric is basically a hormone deficiency state, its symptoms can be reduced by using hormone (estrogen) replacement therapy. Or, when hormone therapy is not suitable or not wanted, by treating the individual symptoms.

Hormone replacement therapy

Estrogen is given in small doses to prevent or relieve menopausal symptoms. Some doctors believe that it should be given for the rest of the woman's life. Others use it only for a year or so, tapering off the doses to make the change gradual. Others won't use it at all. It will not correct pre-existing emotional problems, but women using it tend to have a feeling of well-being and seem to cope more easily with the physical changes. Progestogen may be given as well as estrogen.

Side effects occur in some women. They include nausea, headaches, breast soreness, uterine bleeding, blood clotting, fibroids growing, and diabetic and liver difficulties. They are not very common, but must be watched for. The biggest fear is that of cancer; not because hormone therapy might cause it (short-term therapy probably does not) but because bleeding thought to be due to the treatment might in fact be due to cancer, yet be ignored.

Many doctors prescribe hormone replacement therapy only after doing an endometrial biopsy or a curettage to check that the endometrium is normal. After this, they like to see the woman every six months for a pelvic examination, and for urine and blood pressure checks.

Relief of individual symptoms

- Hot flushes can be helped by clonidine (Dixarit) or belladona (Bellergal) tablets.
- Vaginal and vulval problems, by estrogen creams or by acid jelly.
- Prolapse and urinary problems, by physiotherapy and surgery.
- Tiredness, insomnia, and emotional problems often get better when the other symptoms improve.

Good diet, understanding people, and less physical work help. Tranquilizers usually are not necessary, but they do help some people. Sedatives, at night, may be useful for a while.

Women having menopausal symptoms should consult their family physician or gynecologist. Medication may or may not be required or necessary but often just discussing the symptoms will relieve anxieties and tension which compound the other problems. Estrogen replacement therapy is sometimes used but on an individual case basis.

7
Breast examination

Regular self-examination of the breasts should be performed by every woman over the age of twenty-five years.
It should be done every month, in the week following
menstruation. This time is best because then any premenstrual fullness and discomfort has settled. After the
menopause, the woman should choose a date that is
easy to remember, such as the first of each month, and
continue with regular self-examinations.

Technique of breast self-examination

Looking at the breasts (Figure 7.1a):

- Sit or stand in front of a mirror, in a good light.
- Keep the arms relaxed by the sides.
- Look for changes in the size and shape of the breasts
  and nipples.
- Look for dimpling or puckering of the skin.
- Raise the arms above the head and look at the breasts
  and nipples again.

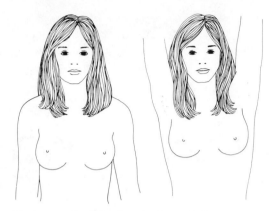

Figure 7.1a Breast self-examination – looking at the breasts

Feeling the breasts (Figure 7.1b):

- Lie down with a small pillow or folded towel under the left shoulder.
- Lift up the left arm.
- Using the right hand, examine the left breast.
- Using the flats (not the tips) of the fingers, work over the whole breast, starting at the armpit and working around.
- Lower the left arm and feel the armpit area again, with the arm lying alongside the body.
- Change the pillow or towel to the other shoulder, and examine the right breast with the left arm.
- Note anything unusual, any thickness or lumps, and go to the doctor straight away if there is anything at all abnormal.

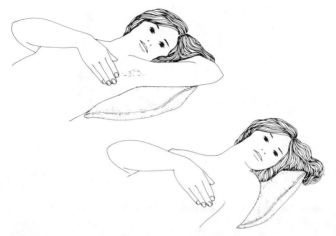

Figure 7.1b Breast self-examination – feeling the breasts

Most breast lumps are not cancer, and the ones that are can often be cured, but only if they are discovered and treated *early*.

Breast cancer

Breast cancer is one of the common cancers in women today. Most at risk are those who:

- Have a family history of breast cancer.
- Have not had children.
- Have cancer of the other breast or endometrium.
- Are in an older age group (especially around meno-pause).

If discovered and treated early, nine out of ten breast cancers have extremely good survival rates. But cancer of the breast often spreads soon after a lump is discovered. That is why doctors don't wait until a "convenient" time before investigating a breast lump. They must never be ignored, because the later stages have poor survival rates.

8
Hospitals and operations

Most hospitals issue information booklets to their patients on admission. These tell about meal times, visiting hours, payment of accounts, and other details of hospital life, and they save people from asking a lot of questions. But few places give much information about what might be involved in the way of preparations and treatments in hospital; the little details that go to make up the whole experience.

Doctors and nurses are usually very happy to explain what they are doing and why, but sometimes they don't remember to explain in advance. Yet it is the procedures that are so routine to them (because they do them every day), that can seem to be so unusual, perhaps unnecessary, so very embarrassing and sometimes even frightening to the woman who doesn't understand what is going on. Of course, not all of the following points apply to every gynecological operation.

Before the operation

Consent for surgery

As well as the routine consent, for those operations that will result in the woman being unable to have more children, some hospitals may require that a special form be signed by both the husband and wife.

Tests

URINE TESTING

This is done routinely, mainly to screen for unsuspected diabetes. A "mid-stream" specimen may also be collected, to be sent to the laboratory for examination for the presence of infection. Urinary infection could cause much discomfort and difficulty after the operation.

CHEST X RAYS

These are sometimes done if there might be chest problems. Lung problems can cause difficulty with general anesthetics or with breathing comfort after the operation.

BLOOD TESTS

These are carried out to check the hemoglobin (iron) level, and to match blood for transfusion if there is expected to be bleeding during the operation. For example, the test would be performed before a hysterectomy but not usually for a tubal ligation.

Other procedures

VAGINAL EXAMINATION

This is often made as a final check for infection and previous clinical findings. Existing infection could spread during the operation or flare up afterwards. A sample of any discharge is sent away for testing.

SHAVING

This is done because hairs naturally harbour organisms. For abdominal operations the area from above the navel to the pubic bone is shaved. For vaginal surgery, a full vulval shave is done, including the pubic hair and the hair on the upper thighs. Some doctors do not require a woman to be shaved before a curette; others do.

ENEMAS

These wash out the lower bowel to prevent contamination during operation. An empty bowel is also much more comfortable during the first few days after a pelvic operation. For the smaller operations a rectal suppository is given instead. The bowel preparation is usually given the night before surgery.

Anesthetist's visit

The doctor responsible for the anesthetic will visit to make sure that there will be no unsuspected difficulties during the operation. The doctor will ask questions about general health, tablets taken, and known allergies. He or she will explain about fasting for a certain number of hours before the operation, and about premedication (usually an injection) given about an hour before surgery to help to dry up secretions and cause relaxation and drowsiness.

Preparing for the operating room

The nurse will supply a special nightgown, hat, and sometimes boots and explain how to put them on. She will put tape around a wedding ring so that it does not slip off and get lost. Any other rings or jewellery should be removed earlier and locked away. All hairpins are taken out and hair is tucked underneath the cap. Any artificial teeth are usually taken out at this stage, although in some places the anesthetist prefers to do this in the operating room. Contact lenses are always re-moved and left in a safe place. After all this, the pre-medication is given and the hour of waiting is spent getting drowsy.

After the operation

Many hospitals have special recovery rooms as part of their operating department. The patient is kept in the recovery room until she is fully conscious, and her pulse, blood pressure, and bandaging are checked regularly. When all is normal, she is taken back to her bed.

Early post-operative routines

These include frequent checking of the pulse, blood pressure, and wound site, and frequent requests to do deep breathing, coughing, and leg movements.

Drips and tubes

Many people are frightened when they wake up from an operation to find an intravenous drip attached to one arm, or bottles and bags attached to the bed to collect urine and wound drainage.

INTRAVENOUS DRIPS
These are used for any of the following reasons:
- If blood has been lost at operation and fluid needs to be replaced.
- If normal eating and drinking will not be resumed for a few days.
- To keep the vein open until the danger of bleeding has passed, usually for about 24 hours (this is routine).

CATHETERS

Catheters, draining the bladder, are used when it would be difficult or painful to pass urine normally. They relieve pressure on the operation site and are usually not felt when in place. They are routine for the first few days after a hysterectomy, vaginal repair, and vulval surgery. Tablets to prevent infection may be prescribed when a catheter is in.

WOUND DRAINS

Wound drains take excess blood and fluid away from the operation site to enable it to heal more quickly. Sometimes they drain directly into the dressings (pads and bandages), and sometimes they are connected to a bottle or bag attached to the bed.

Vulval washdowns

Vulval washdowns are done routinely after operations which are followed by blood drainage from the vagina. They prevent infection and make the area much more comfortable, until the woman is able to shower.

Ray lamps

These are often used after a perineorrhaphy (often done as part of a vaginal repair). Because the perineum is in such a moist dark area, the light and warmth provided by the lamp helps the wound to heal quickly. The lamp treatment usually starts several days after the operation. Salt baths may be used as well.

Removal of stitches

Abdominal wounds may be closed with clips or stitches. These are usually removed before the patient goes home;

it depends on the size and site of the wound. Usually every second stitch or clip is removed on one day, and the remainder the following day. Vaginal wounds are usually closed with self-dissolving stitches that fall out by themselves on about the ninth or tenth day. When this happens it is often accompanied by a slight odourless yellowish discharge, which may take a few weeks to disappear completely. If the discharge becomes smelly or increases, it should be reported.

Going home

Before leaving hospital the woman should make sure that she knows exactly what to do to fully recover and prevent problems. She should know when and how to take prescribed tablets or do treatments, how to look after the wound, when she should next see the doctor, when she may go back to work, how much lifting or housework is allowed, when to resume sexual intercourse, and whether or not her former method of family planning is still suitable.

Gynecological operations have, for all sorts of reasons, been given an air of mystery and fear. An operation need not be a dreadful experience; it can be regarded positively, as something that will relieve annoying symptoms or prevent disorders from becoming worse.

Common gynecological operations – useful guidelines

Operation	What is done/ taken out	What is left (specific)	Effect on body-functioning	Physical effect on sexual activity (once healed)
Total abdominal hysterectomy	uterus (including cervix)	ovaries vagina	no more periods; if premeno-pausal, will not have a sudden climacteric	nil
Total abdominal hysterectomy with bilateral salpingo-oophorectomy	uterus tubes ovary	vagina	climacteric will result, possibly with symptoms; no more periods; estrogen replacement may be ordered	estrogen withdrawal; dryness etc, otherwise nil
Radical abdominal hysterectomy, Bilateral salpingo-oophorectomy & Bilateral pelvic node dissection (Wertheim's hysterectomy)	uterus tubes ovaries; upper third of vagina; pelvic lymph nodes	lower vagina	will have climacteric, menopause; no estrogen replacement given	shortness of vagina is not main problem if op preceded by radiation treatment, could be contraction, also lack of secretions (estrogen withdrawal)
Myomectomy	fibroids shelled out from uterus	uterus and all other reproductive organs	nil	nil

Effect on reproductive ability	Will there be a scar?	Special things to expect after the operation	Will there be vaginal blood loss?	Days in hospital (approx)
ceased	yes – lower abdominal	IV drip; wound drain tubes; possibly a urinary catheter (3–5 days)	yes	10–14
ceased	yes – lower abdominal	IV drip; wound drains; possibly a urinary catheter for 3–5 days	yes	10–14
ceased	yes – lower abdominal	IV drip; wound drains through a tube; urinary catheter 3–5 days	yes	14–21
retained; often improved; labour closely supervised	yes – lower abdominal	possibly wound drains	probably	7–10

Operation	What is done/ taken out	What is left (specific)	Effect on body-functioning	Physical effect on sexual activity (once healed)
Abdominal tubal ligation	tubes cut; 2.5 cm removed from each; ends tied separately	uterus ovaries vagina	nil	nil
Ovarian cystectomy	cyst tissue removed from ovary, but remaining ovarian tissue conserved	uterus tubes vagina some ovarian tissue	nil	nil
Oophorectomy	ovary(ies) removed	uterus vagina	if unilateral – nil; if bilateral – climacteric will occur; no more periods	nil, if unilateral; estrogen withdrawal effects if bilateral
Ventro-suspension	round ligaments shortened to hold uterus forward	everything	nil	nil
Examination under anesthesia (EUA)	vaginal (pelvic) examination under anesthetic	everything	nil	nil
Dilatation and curettege (D & C)	cervix gradually dilated; lining of uterus scraped	everything	nil	nil

Effect on reproductive ability	Will there be a scar?	Special things to expect after the operation	Will there be vaginal blood loss?	Days in hospital (approx)
ceased	yes – small lower abdominal	–	possibly	5–10
retained	yes – lower abdominal	–	possibly	7–10
if bilateral – ceased	yes – lower abdominal	depends on indication for operation; in itself, possibly only wound drainage	possibly	7–10
nil	yes – small, lower abdominal	–	possibly	7–10
nil	no	–	no	*0–2
retained	no	nil	yes	*0–2

*0 days = done as outpatient in some centres.

Operation	What is done/ taken out	What is left (specific)	Effect on body-functioning	Physical effect on sexual activity (once healed)
Bartholin's marsupial-ization	Bartholin's gland opened and edges sewn to vaginal wall thus creating a pouch or channel for drainage	everything	nil	improvement of lubrication
Vulvectomy 1 simple	labia majora, minora and clitoris	urethral orifice and vagina	nil	still capable of intercourse but different, because clitoris absent
2 radical	whole vulva including skin and fat above pubis and groin lymph glands	urethral orifice and vagina	chronic edema of legs is common	younger women should be capable of intercourse; vaginal delivery has been reported after this operation
Vaginal repairs Colporrhaphy	nothing removed; cutting into vaginal wall and sewing it more firmly to strengthen it	everything	nil	still possible; may improve/ worsen difficulties

Effect on reproductive ability	Will there be a scar?	Special things to expect after the operation	Will there be vaginal blood loss?	Days in hospital (approx)
retained	small pouch opening into vagina; not obvious	small pack in 48 hours	some drainage after pack out	3–7
retained	yes (vulval)	urinary catheter 3–5 days	possibly wound drainage	5–7
retained	yes, vulval and lower abdominal	IV drip; urinary catheter; closed suction wound drainage; raw wound – skin grafting possible	wound drainage	3–12 weeks
retained; second stage of labour closely observed	not obvious (inside vagina)	possibly an IV drip; urinary catheter 3–5 days; pack in vagina for 24 hrs; stitches will dissolve 9–10 days – yellowish discharge	yes	7–14

Operation	What is done/ taken out	What is left (specific)	Effect on body-functioning	Physical effect on sexual activity (once healed)
Manchester repair	uterus lifted up by shortening supporting ligaments; vaginal part of cervix removed; front and back vaginal walls repaired	everything but vaginal portion of cervix	nil	as for vaginal repair
Vaginal hysterectomy and repair	vaginal wall opened; uterus removed via vagina; vaginal walls repaired	ovaries vagina	no more periods; will not have artificial climacteric	as for vaginal repair
Laparoscopy	direct inspection of pelvic contents through hollow tube (laparoscope)	everything	nil	nil
Vaginal urethroplasty	tissue around urethra reinforced by stitching to support urethra	everything	nil	as for vaginal repair
Sling operations (Marshall-Marchetti)	elevation and support of bladder neck by fixing it to the back of the symphysis pubis	everything	nil	nil

Effect on reproductive ability	Will there be a scar?	Special things to expect after the operation	Will there be vaginal blood loss?	Days in hospital (approx)
fertility may be lowered because less cervical mucus will be produced; otherwise, as for vaginal repair	not obvious (inside vagina)	as for vaginal repair	yes	10–14
ceased	not obvious (inside vagina)	as for vaginal repair	yes	10–14
retained unless diathermy used specifically to occlude tubes	one or two tiny incisions near umbilicus (band-aids)	nursed flat for 8 hours	possibly	1–2
retained as for vaginal repair	not obvious (inside vagina)	possibly an IV drip; possibly a vaginal pack; catheter 3–5 days; usually no voiding problems afterwards	possibly wound drainage	10–14
retained	small, lower abdominal	as above	no	10–14

1 2 3 4 5   143404   88 87 86 85 84